Cannabis Concepts:

A Guide to Making and Using Cannabis Oil at Home

This guide is intended for those who have **already decided** to use cannabis.

The contents outline different methods of making and using cannabis oils. It explains the why behind the how.

At its best, this guide will empower the reader to make and use cannabis oils at home with confidence. Each person can determine for themselves what makes sense. **There is no right or wrong way to make or use cannabis!**

There is a lot of technical information explained in a clear, concise way. All of the concepts overlap. It is best to briefly read, or skim, the entire manual before attempting to understand each section on its own. It is important to get the big picture before understanding one word or idea. If a concept or word does not make sense, including the Vocabulary and FAQ's at the beginning, keep reading and come back to it later,

This is by no means an exhaustive guide, just an introduction to key concepts.

**Although the concepts apply to oils used for inhaling, this guide is meant for those using cannabis orally or topically.

ISBN 978-1-950602-00-1

Published by Retrograde Books
Printed in the U.S.A.

RxBooks

Welcome,

When I decided to use cannabis to treat our child's epilepsy, I researched and experimented with growing and making cannabis oils at home. At the time there were not many options in the dispensaries even though we lived in a legal state. I was wanting what I thought was the perfect medicine and would make it myself.

After much experimentation, research, and anecdotal evidence from parents around the world, I realized there was no perfect solution, but that all cannabis is useful in different ways. I wrote this guide in an attempt to simplify a subject that has become increasingly complex.

This guide is intended to help readers understand basic cannabis concepts. Using common household items, anyone can make their own remedies. Repeat: Each person can determine for themselves what makes sense. There is no right or wrong way to make or use cannabis!

I am not a doctor nor do I claim to be one. I am a mom. That's it. The content is purely opinion and should not be taken as medical advice. Everyone is responsible for themselves. Thank goodness.

Angie

Table of Contents

Vocabulary

Cannabis: Scientific name for marijuana, weed, pot, ganja, hemp, etc.

Cannabis Oil: Oil found in the *trichomes* of the cannabis plant. When extracted, this oil is a sticky resin. It is usually mixed with a *carrier oil* which is also called "Cannabis Oil". One is **pure** (see *FECO*), and one is **diluted**.

Cannabinoid: A medicinal chemical component of cannabis that interacts with the body. Usually abbreviated with 3-4 letter acronyms (ex: THC, CBD, THCA)

CBD (Cannabidiol): A non-psychoactive cannabinoid found in cannabis. Found in hemp and other types of cannabis. Most studied in children with intractable seizures.

CBD Oil: Cannabis Oil that has a large amount of CBD. If it has less than .3% THC, it can be called Hemp Oil. (See *Hemp Oil* for clarification)

Carrier Oil: An oil or fat added to pure cannabis oil (resin) or infused. Cannabinoids are fat soluble and seem to absorb into the body better with a fat.[1]
Ex: coconut oil, fractionated coconut (MCT) oil, butter, olive oil.

Decarboxylate (decarb): Heating cannabis flower or extract to speed up the natural chemical process of decomposition. This process changes the cannabinoid profile.

Edible: Food containing cannabis. Typically desserts or gummies.

FECO or RSO: "Rick Simpson Oil" (RSO) is a common term for cannabis oil extracted from the plant using a solvent. Rick Simpson is a cannabis oil pioneer and cancer survivor who popularized using cannabis to cure cancer. To avoid legal arguments, "Full Extract Cannabis Oil", or FECO, is the current industry lingo for cannabis oil extracted with a solvent. Pure cannabis oil (no carrier oil).

Hash: Only the tips of the *trichomes*.

---

[1] Priyamveda, Sharva. "Chemistry, Metabolism, and Toxicology of Cannabis" 2012 Fall 7(4) 149-156
https://www.ncbi.nlm.nih.gov/pmc/articles/PMC3570572/

Hemp: *Legally* any cannabis plant that contains less than .3% THC . **Historically** a cannabis variety grown for fiber and seeds.

Hemp oil: Any cannabis oil less than .3% THC. Typically high CBD content.

Hemp seed oil: Oil made from pressing *cannabis (hemp)* **seeds**. NOT the same as hemp oil made from the **resin** from trichomes of the plant. Does not contain cannabinoids.

Isolate: One cannabinoid removed from cannabis oil. Usually CBD or THC.

Kief: Similar to hash but has more plant material because it is collected in a slightly different manner.

Raw Cannabis: Flower, hash or extract that has not been heated. Freshly harvested. Many cannabinoids are in acid form (see chart p.14). Ex: THCA or CBDA.

Solvent: Liquid that dissolves, or extracts, cannabis resin from the plant. Examples: grain alcohol, isopropyl alcohol (ISO), butane (BHO), liquid CO_2.

THC (Tetrahydrocannabinol): Most popular cannabinoid. Psychoactive creating a "high" when ingested or inhaled. There are several different THC cannabinoids but THC-9 or delta-9 is the cannabinoid this book refers to.

Trichome: Small hair-like follicle on the cannabis plant containing resin, or oil. Cannabis has **glandular** trichomes, meaning the glands extend into the leaves and stems. Non-glandular trichomes do not penetrate the plant (ex: tomato plant).

Terpenes: Fragrant chemical component found in plants responsible for smell. Terpenes are also medicinal.[2] A cannabis strain has a terpene profile in addition to a cannabinoid profile.   Terpenes are the main component of essential oils.

Topical: Cannabis product used on the skin.

Whole plant extract: Cannabis oil extracted, or infused, without removing or adding any additional chemical components (cannabinoids or terpenes).

---

[2] Nuttinen, J. "Medicinal Properties of Terpenes Found in Cannabis Sativa". Eur J Med Chem 2018 Sept 5;157 198-228 https://www.ncbi.nlm.nih.gov/pubmed/30096653

FAQS

Why make oil? Why not just smoke cannabis?

Extracting cannabis oil concentrates the cannabinoids and terpenes to make a more potent medicine.

One of my teachers had cancer for years and smoked for years. Although it helped ease her pain and discomfort, it was not until she started taking full extract oil that her bone density increased, her tumor shrunk, and her cancer evaporated.

Oil is a more practical way to dose children, elderly, medically frail, and anyone else wishing to avoid smoking.

Will I get high?

If the product has THC, it is likely you will feel a change in your mental state. This may mean elation, relief, anxiety, an altered state of mind. How "high" depends on how much you consume and your tolerance level. It is possible to increase tolerance so feeling the effects will not be as likely.

If the product does not contain THC, it most likely contains CBD. You will most likely not feel any significant mental changes but may feel relief.

Can I become addicted?

Cannabis can be as addictive as any other substance and is best used in a protocol while the root of the problem is addressed. This includes depression, anxiety, pain, and other ailments. CBD is currently used to help those addicted, recover.[3]

Can I treat my pet with cannabis?

Cannabis for pets is a growing industry. Consider the size of the animal when dosing and whether the supplement contains THC or CBD and how much. A weaker topical high CBD remedy is a good place to start.

---

[3] Shannon, Scott. "Cannabidiol for Decreasing Addictive Use of Marijuana. Integ Med 2015 Dec 14(6) 31-35. https://www.ncbi.nlm.nih.gov/pmc/articles/PMC4718203/

Where do I start?

Begin with the easiest solution. This may be growing and making your own, buying a syringe of full extract oil and diluting it on your own, buying flower and making your own oil, or just walking into a dispensary and buying something off the shelves depending on the laws in your location. As far as use, a topical remedy may be a good place to start.

Will Cannabis interact negatively with my other medications?

Many cannabinoids are processed in the liver **p450 cytochrome system**. Different cytochromes process different cannabinoids. If your medication is also processed in the liver, it may increase or decrease the effects of the medication or the cannabis. [4]

Taking cannabis 4-8 hours apart from other oral medications is usually recommended. Using a sublingual dosing may also avoid negative drug interactions.

How do I use cannabis for my condition?

See **Methods of Delivery p.30**. Consider the cannabinoids but also where and how the body is affected. Several methods can be used to fully address a condition.

In general, if the condition is related to nerves or the nervous system, inflammation, depression or anxiety, try higher CBD products. If the condition is physical or mental tension, nausea or cancer, try THC products. Each individual responds differently to strains and methods of delivery. Experiment for best results.

Will Cannabis help my condition?

Cannabis is considered an "adaptogen" in herbal medicine. Meaning it is able to **adapt** to the body's needs. Finding the right combination of strain and dose may take time. Cannabis does help many individuals with a variety of conditions. However, cannabis does not help everyone.

Cannabis is best used in a treatment plan that addresses all aspects of the body, mind, and spirit.

---

[4] https://www.projectcbd.org/science/cannabis-pharmacology/cbd-drug-interactions-role-cytochrome-p450
Jiang, R. "Identification of cytochrome p450 enzymes responsible for metabolism of cannabidiol" Life Sci 2011 Aug 1. 29(5-6) https://www.ncbi.nlm.nih.gov/pubmed/21704641

Parts of a Cannabis Plant

It is useful to know a little about the cannabis plant and how it grows in order to understand how to make cannabis oil.

Cannabis is Dioecious, meaning there are separate male and female plants.

Cannabis oil is produced in *glandular trichomes*, small hairlike follicles that extend into the flowers, leaves, and stems. Male plants do not produce many trichomes, and therefore, oil. Female plants have flowers and produce more trichomes when they are not fertilized (seeded). Growers use a method called *sinsemilla*, growing only **female plants** to produce the most trichomes and oil. The majority of the trichomes are located on the flowers (or buds) of the female plants.

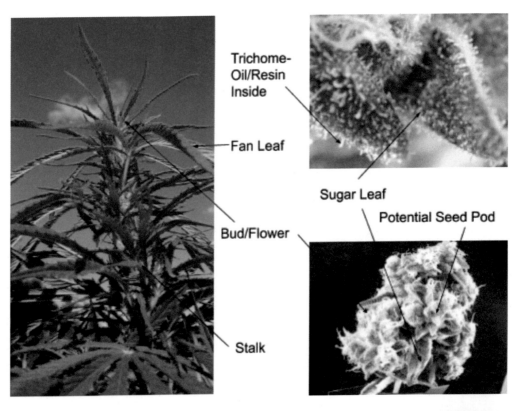

Trichome-
Oil/Resin
Inside

Fan Leaf

Sugar Leaf

Potential Seed Pod

Bud/Flower

Stalk

Industrial hemp is grown for seeds and stalks. Both male and female plants are grown and pollination occurs.

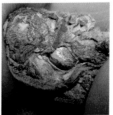

What is Cannabis? Hemp? Marijuana?

Cannabis is the scientific name (preferred reference for legalization)
Marijuana is a common name for cannabis with THC and getting "high" (pot, weed, etc)
Hemp is a variety (strains) of cannabis containing less than .3% THC and high CBD

GENOTYPE

Kingdom-Plant
Family-Cannabaceae
Genus-Cannabis
SubSpecies-C. Sativa, C. Indica, C. Ruderalis
Variety=Strains

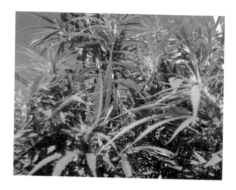

Hemp Confusion

Historically, *"industrial hemp"* is a variety of cannabis bred and used for its **stalks and seeds**. It was widely used in the early 1900's as a source of fiber, fuel, building materials, among other things. Currently, hemp seeds and **hemp seed oil** are popular products of industrial hemp. Both male and female plants are grown.

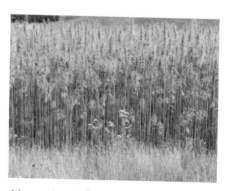

Hemp bred for seeds and stalks.

Legally, *"hemp"* is defined as cannabis containing less than .3% THC. When it was rediscovered that cannabis oil with high levels of CBD helped children with seizures, the industry began calling this "hemp oil" in order to grow and sell it legally. This cannabis originally had higher THC but was bred over time to have less than .3% to meet the legal requirements. It is often marketed as "CBD oil". This hemp is bred for trichomes (resin) and only female plants are grown.

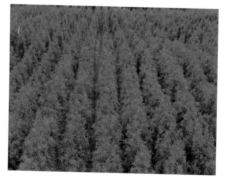

Hemp bred for resin.

All hemp is CBD oil but not all CBD is hemp. It must have <.3% to be labeled and sold as hemp.

Choosing a Strain to Grow or Use

For beginners, start with something easy to obtain that contains the initial desired cannabinoids. **All cannabis contains medicinal components.** Even if it is only one choice, begin there.

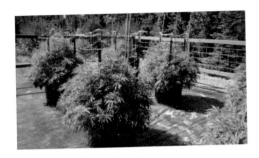

For those in legal locations with many choices, test a few options to see how your body reacts. Use different strains but try to use a whole plant extract. Each individual plant, has a unique combination of nature and nurture that may produce different results.

It is common to switch strains when one does not seem to "work" anymore. See Dosing p.33.

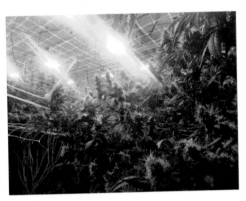

Strains are often discussed strictly by their **genotype, Indica or Sativa**. It is often explained Sativa produces a "mind high" and an Indica produces a "body high". Or that one is preferable to the other in certain medical conditions. However, with intense crossbreeding and hybridization over the past several decades, it is difficult to currently class a strain in this way. Even if a pure (landrace strain) Sativa or Indica is used, an individual responds uniquely.

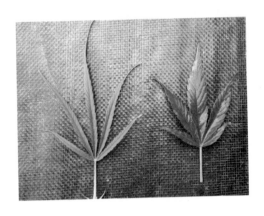

Seeking heirloom (landrace) strains may interest those who also seek heirloom tomatoes, apples, roses, etc. for the same reasons. An older, developed strain tends to have easily replicated effects and years of trial on its side. Again, nurture is the other half of the equation.

More common, with the introduction of testing, is choosing a strain based on chemotype, or chemical composition.

Cannabinoid Profile (Chemotype)

Each strain has a unique fingerprint of cannabinoids and terpenes, or chemotype. They all work together to create an effect in the body.

How each plant is grown, harvested, and decarbed can affect this profile.

This photo shows the main cannabinoids present in 5 different flower samples. THC and CBD are currently the two most discussed cannabinoids. Each strain has one or the other, or a combination.

Although *all* **cannabinoids (over 100) add to the effect of cannabis**, it is useful, and common, to discuss and choose a product based on the amount of THC or CBD in it.

If scientific evidence is important to you, look up the condition you are treating. New studies occur daily. If you prefer anecdotal evidence, it is abundant both on the internet and in life.

A few guidelines I find useful:

If the condition is nerve related (nervous system), inflammation, anxiety, depression or autism, try higher CBD.

If the condition is tension of mind or body (muscles), cancer, nausea or ADHD, try higher THC.

If working with a child, try higher CBD or a mix.

For insomnia, try older dried or cured cannabis which contains a different chemotype than a freshly harvested product.

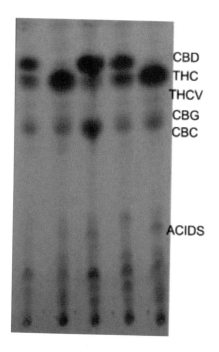

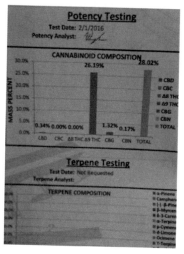

What is Decarboxylation? Why?

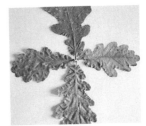

After harvest, cannabinoids continue to change during **decomposition**. Chemically, the acid cannabinoids lose a "**carboxyl**" group (COOH) and release carbon dioxide. This process is also known as **decarboxylation**.

All things in nature lose molecules as they decompose. In food, this prepares it to be more easily digested by the body. For example, milk is fermented into yogurt or kefir, cabbage into sauerkraut or kimchi, meat into sausage, flour into sourdough.

The same concept is true for cannabis. A product that has been cured, or decarbed is typically more easily digested, or used, by the body.

The best example of how decarboxylation affects the body is THCA changing to THC. Raw (freshly harvested) cannabis has mostly THCA and very little THC. THCA is non-psychoactive. However, when decarbed, it turns into THC, the common psychoactive. See photo p.16.

When smoking, decarboxylation occurs when lighting the material on fire. When making oils, the material needs to be heated in another way, or cured over time.

Curing allows the cannabis to naturally decarboxylate over time. In the same way vegetables are fermented, connoisseurs cure flower in a mason jar, "burping" it occasionally to release the carbon dioxide that is created as it decarbs. After 3-6 months, it will have converted around 50% of its acid cannabinoids. The flower remains moist so it is not harsh when smoking. However, when making oil, the condition of the flower is not as important. A dry flower is still useful for making oil. Some people are using raw (acid only) oils, attempting to stop the curing process. In my personal experience, many of the THCA continue the curing process into THC. (CBDA stays an acid longer because it has a higher decarb temp point).

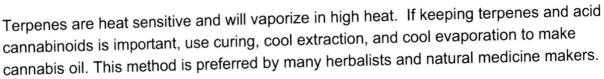

Terpenes are heat sensitive and will vaporize in high heat. If keeping terpenes and acid cannabinoids is important, use curing, cool extraction, and cool evaporation to make cannabis oil. This method is preferred by many herbalists and natural medicine makers.

Most studies and anecdotal evidence is based on fully decarbed cannabis. This requires heating with an external source. Heating the cannabis can happen **before** (heated in an oven as flower), **during** (heated evaporation), or **after** (heated as either FECO or a diluted oil) the extraction process.

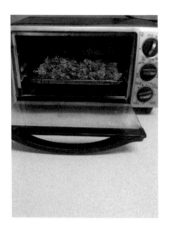 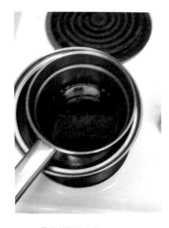 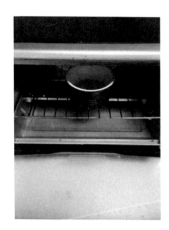

BEFORE   **DURING**   **AFTER**

For beginners, decarbing flower in an oven ahead of time is recommended.

How decarboxylation occurs *can slightly influence* the cannabinoid content. However, for beginners and at-home oil makers, this is not something to be overly obsessed with. In general, a longer, gentler decarb process will produce slightly higher cannabinoid content. Several gadgets are sold for this purpose.

CANNABIS DECARBOXYLATION TIMES (APPROXIMATE)
***Too high will burn off cannabinoids, too low will not convert. **250F/120C is a MAXIMUM.**
Cannabis is forgiving in heat compared to other herbs. Decarb begins around 170F/65C but for a full decarb in a shorter time the temperature needs to be in this range.

Temp in F	Temp in C	Minutes
250	120	25
240	115	35
230	110	45
220	104	55
210	99	65

How Cannabinoids Change in a Plant Over Time

The cannabinoids present in cannabis change throughout the life cycle of the plant. All cannabinoids begin as an "acid" chemical and slowly change as the plant grows, is harvested, and decomposes (decarbs). There are over 100 named and unnamed cannabinoids at the time of this writing. However, only a few are present in amounts greater than 1%. The following chart shows a few common cannabinoids and how they change over time. **Sometimes a cannabinoid is present because of its genetics (nature) and sometimes it is present because of how it is grown (nurture) or processed.**

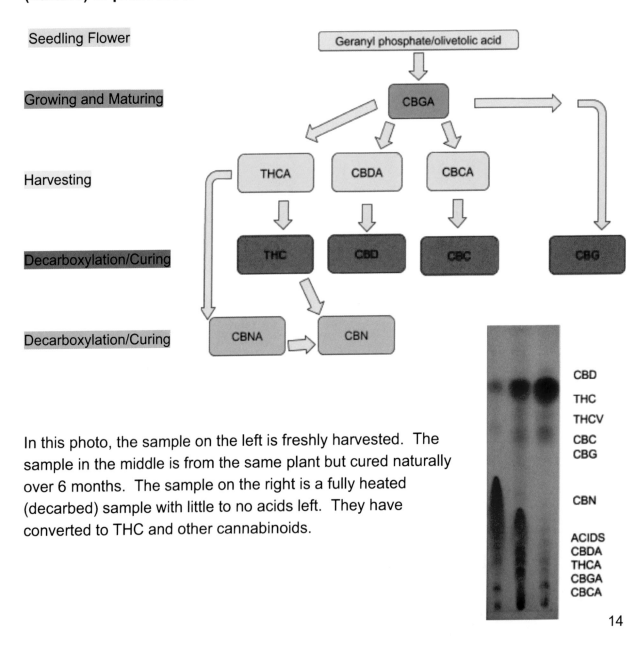

In this photo, the sample on the left is freshly harvested. The sample in the middle is from the same plant but cured naturally over 6 months. The sample on the right is a fully heated (decarbed) sample with little to no acids left. They have converted to THC and other cannabinoids.

14

Methods of Extraction

Now that the basics of cannabis have been explored, the following methods will make more sense.

There are several ways to separate cannabis oil from the flower: extract the cannabis oil (solvent), infuse the cannabis oil, remove the tips of the trichomes (hash), or press the oil out (rosin). Whether at home or in a production facility, the basic concepts are the same. **All methods are whole plant extracts.**

	PROS	CONS
Solvent (Alcohol)	Full extraction using all resin in plant Most potent with ability to dilute as needed	Bitter taste, especially sublingual
Infusion (Oil / Butter)	Easiest method Directly extracted into oil	Least potent Most smell
Hash / Kief	Little to no smell Kief is very easy	Uses only part of trichome leaving much more resin inside plant
Rosin	Solventless. Pure oil after pressing	Difficult to reproduce consistently.

The Rosin method uses high heat and pressure to squeeze cannabis oil out of the trichomes. I find this method difficult to use and mix with a carrier oil after the extraction. This method is not explored in detail in this guide.

There is no "right" way to make oil. Any combination of time, temperature, movement, and appliances is effective. Beginners tend to get overwhelmed so the following pages provide specific instructions which are free to be manipulated as needed.

Ingredients

The following are what I use based on my current beliefs and situation. **Use what makes sense and is easy.**

Cannabis:

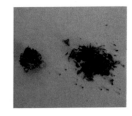

Cannabis flower has the most trichomes, therefore oil.
Trim also contain oil but slightly less than flower.
Fan leaves and stems also have oil but about ¼ the amount.

Alcohol:

I prefer 95% grain alcohol (ex: Everclear) for its efficiency in extracting and reclaiming.
It does leave a bitter residue which can be difficult to tolerate in sublingual use.
Any alcohol will work, vodka, rum, whiskey, etc. Use highest proof available.
Some people ask about Isopropyl Alcohol and my recommendation is **food grade** Isopropyl. Not rubbing alcohol at the drugstore, although it will extract in the same way.

Oil:

I prefer fractionated coconut oil, also known as MCT (medium chain triglyceride) oil for oral and sublingual use. I use it for many purposes in my home so it is easy for me.
I use virgin coconut oil for topical infusions because I like that it is solid at room temperature. Any oil or fat will work.

Some people ask about **glycerin**. Use it in the same way as an oil (infuse or carrier oil).
I personally find it sticky and irritating to work with so I do not use it.

Extras:

I use local beeswax as an additive to topicals for thickening and skin absorption.
Similar ingredients include cocoa butter, shea butter, etc. I use non-GMO lecithin in oral and sublingual preparation because I believe it increases the effectiveness (bioavailability).

Solvent

Solvents dissolve the "skin" of the trichome and plant matter to access the oil inside the glands. Examples include: Ethanol alcohol, Isopropyl alcohol (ISO), butane (BHO), and liquid CO_2. Alcohol has been used in herbal extractions for thousands of years. Most herbal remedies (and cough syrup) have food grade grain alcohol as the base. **Food grade alcohol is the recommended solvent for beginners.** The higher the proof, the faster the alcohol will extract and then evaporate. This is because there is less water in the alcohol.

Working With Alcohol and Heat

High proof alcohol is flammable.
The higher the percentage the more flammable.
Do not use around open flames. Do not use at high heat.
If using heat for extraction or evaporation,
keep under 212F/100C.

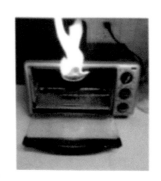

Use common sense. With small batches and little
to no heat, there is little concern. Be aware but not afraid.

0. PAGE 12 DECARB/BLEND THE CANNABIS FLOWER Recommended for beginners

1. SOAK AND SHAKE OR BLEND THE CANNABIS

Reasons vary for different soaking times. If getting the most resin out of the cannabis is the goal, I recommend soaking and shaking or blending for 3-4 hours. Heat during this step helps especially with lower proof alcohol like vodka, but is not necessary. Other variables include blending/shaking and straining.

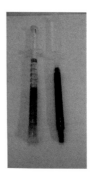

A quick soak (<1min) will extract just the tips of the trichomes. The oil will be much lighter in color like the sample on the left, and similar to oil made from hash. There is still oil remaining in the cannabis.

2. STRAIN THE CANNABIS

After the plant material is soaked several hours, it is strained. The cannabis resin is still in the alcohol. This is called a tincture. Some people prefer to use it in this form.

3. EVAPORATE THE ALCOHOL

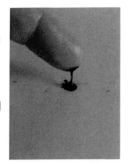

Most common (and my preference) is to remove, or evaporate, the alcohol and mix the remaining **sticky oil** with a carrier oil. Evaporation can be **cool** (air/fan)**, heated** (double broiler), or **distilled** (machine). **Cool evaporation is recommended for beginners.**
As the alcohol evaporates first, the water content is left behind creating small milky puddles. This is normal and will take longer to evaporate. The lower the alcohol proof or percentage, the more water.

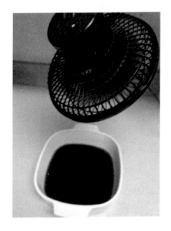
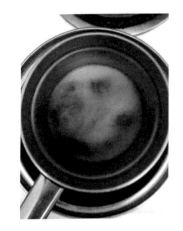
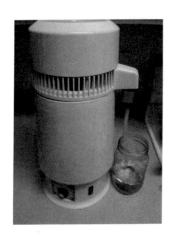

COOL   **HEATED**   **DISTILLED**

Heated evaporation is best done at 212F/100C with a double boiler to avoid burning the cannabis oil at the end.   Turning off the heat and letting the last bit of alcohol to cool evap is also an option for beginners.

Distilling with a machine (as pictured) recovers, or reclaims, the alcohol so it can be used again. See Resources.

4. MIX FECO WITH CARRIER OIL (IF DESIRED)

In larger batches, the oil can be drawn into syringes; but for smaller batches, there is usually only 1-2 ml of FECO and it saves time and oil to mix it during preparation. Mix 20 ml carrier oil to 1 ml FECO. (1oz/30g flower makes approximately 1-2ml FECO).

ALCOHOL COOL EXTRACT / COOL EVAP

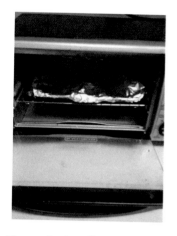

Decarb 1oz/30g Flower

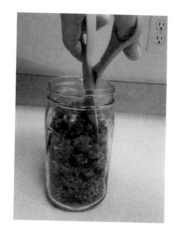

Blend or Cut

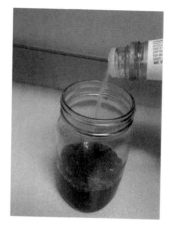

Cover with Alcohol

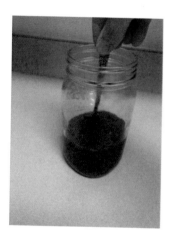

Soak and Stir

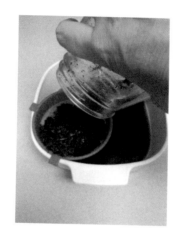

Strain Plant Material

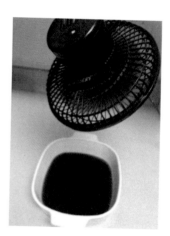

Evaporate

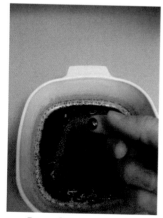

Dry, Sticky Resin
Remains

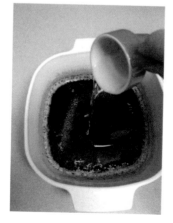

Warm and Add 20ml Oil

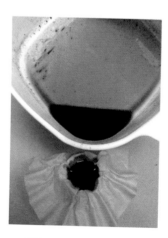

Filter Into Bottle

SOLAR OIL (NO ELECTRICITY)

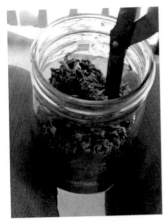

Cut to Reduce Volume

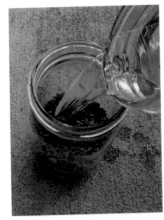

Cover with Alcohol

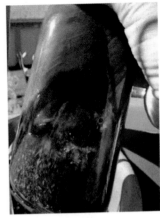

Shake

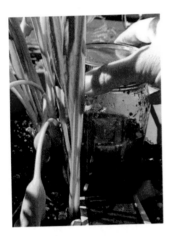

Soak in Sun

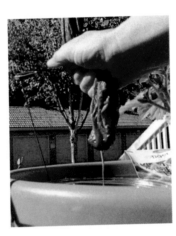

Strain Plant Material

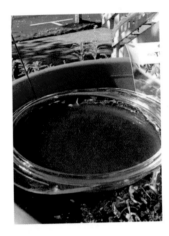

Evaporate in Sun

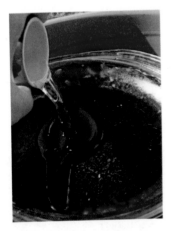

Add Oil to Warm Resin

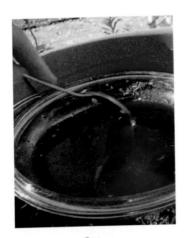

Stir

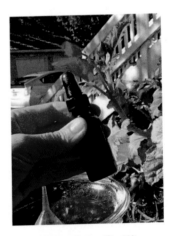

Filter Into Bottle

ALCOHOL HEATED EXTRACT / HEATED EVAP

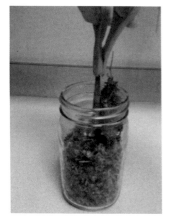

Blend or Cut

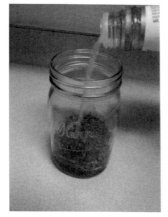

Cover with Alcohol

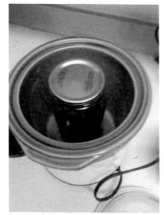

Soak and Stir
in Crockpot

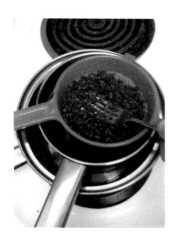

Strain Plant Material

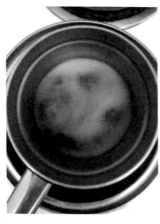

Double Boil Alcohol to
Evaporate

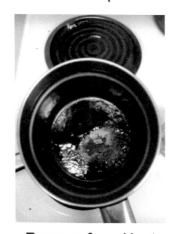

Remove from Heat
Before Burning Resin

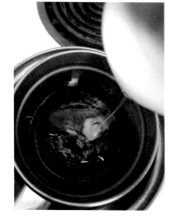

Add Oil to Warm Resin

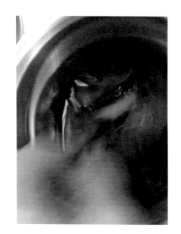

Stir in Carrier Oil

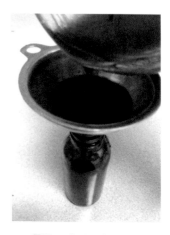

Filter Into Bottle

Infusion

In an infusion, the cannabis flower is soaked directly into the carrier oil (coconut oil, butter, glycerin). Over heat and time, the trichome "skin" is broken down, releasing the resin into the carrier oil. This method is fast and simple. It is not as strong as an alcohol extract (FECO), but double or triple infusing can create a stronger oil if desired.

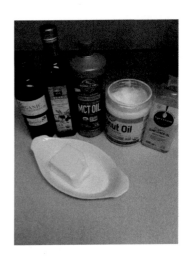

0. PAGE 12 DECARB AND BLEND THE CANNABIS

1. SOAK AND STIR THE CANNABIS

Put the cannabis flower and 1 cup of desired oil in either a crockpot, or a mason jar with lid slightly on the inside of a crockpot if the vessel is too large. . Warm for 2-3 hours. Stir or blend occasionally.

2. STRAIN THE CANNABIS

The plant material is strained and the diluted cannabis oil remains.

For a stronger oil, double or triple infuse the oil. After the first infusion, strain, then add more cannabis flower to the already infused oil.

3. ADD ANY ADDITIONAL INGREDIENTS

For a topical add 1-2oz/30-60g beeswax or cocoa butter depending on desired consistency. Otherwise use as is orally, sublingual, or in a capsule.

CANNABIS OIL INFUSION

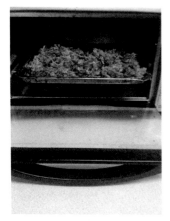

Decarb 1oz/30g Flower

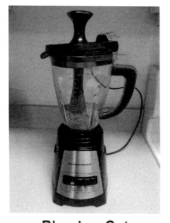

Blend or Cut

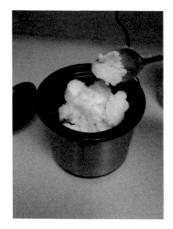

Cover with 1c/240ml Oil

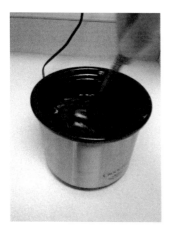

Heat, Soak, and Stir

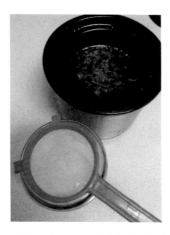

Strain Plant Material

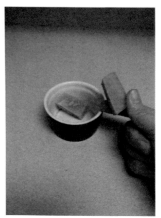

Optional 1oz/30g
Beeswax

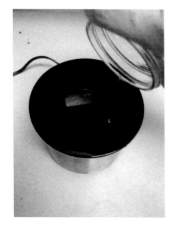

Melt Beeswax into Oil

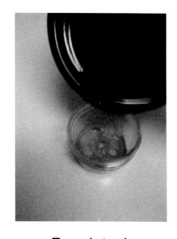

Pour Into Jar

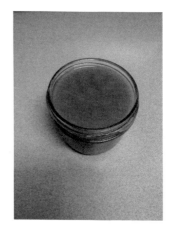

Cool

23

Hash

Hash is the tips of the trichomes. There is still oil left in the glands. Benefits include no smell and a lighter oil which is mild tasting compared to the FECO alcohol method.

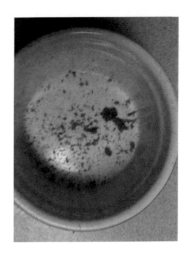

1. PREP BOWL WITH 2 STRAINERS

The first mesh liner is super fine and only allows water to flow through (pillowcase or nut milk bag). The second mesh has larger pores allowing the trichomes to filter through (paint strainer)

Bags are sold online according to pore size, or micron. The smallest size is pore is about 25 (bottom liner) and the largest is 220 (top liner).

2. ADD CANNABIS AND ICE AND WATER

First add cannabis flower in its original form (not blended). Add ice to cover and then cold water. Let sit.

3. GENTLY STIR

After 20 minutes of soaking in the ice water, the trichomes are knocked off by the ice and stirring utensil. Stir for up to 10 minutes.

4. RINSE RINSE RINSE

Lift the bags. The water will run out. Rinse the cannabis thoroughly and allow the trichomes to run into the bottom strainer. Rinse for up to 10 minutes.

5. COLLECT HASH

The hash is collected in the bottom mesh. Rinse into a smaller area of the bag and let dry on the counter. (SEE KIEF p.26 FOR ADDITIONAL INSTRUCTIONS)

ICE WATER HASH (NO SMELL)

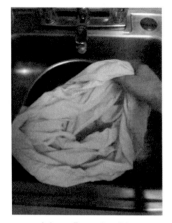

Line Bowl with
Pillowcase

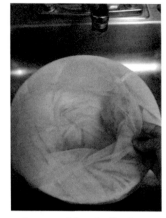

Layer Mesh Paint
Strainer

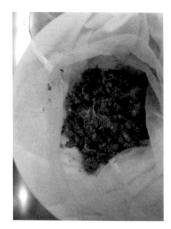

Add 1oz/30g Flower

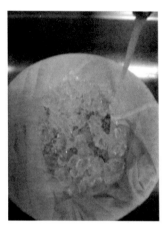

Cover with Ice and
Water, Soak 20 Minutes

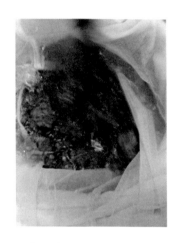

Stir Gently and Rinse

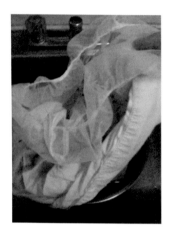

Remove Liners

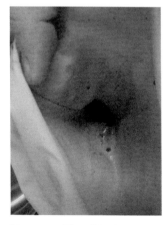

Remove Top Strainer and
Rinse Hash into Corner

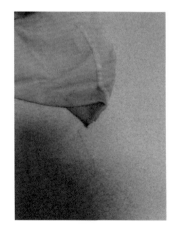

Dry

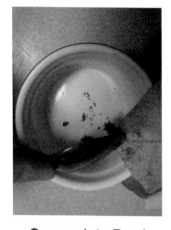

Scrape Into Bowl

Kief

Kief is hash with more plant matter. It is a fast way to get mostly trichomes; but there will be some plant matter and therefore smell if it is heated. There will still be resin in the glands of the plant material.

1. FREEZE CANNABIS FLOWER OVERNIGHT

2. RUB GENTLY OVER MESH STRAINER

A simple mesh strainer or splatter screen work fine. The larger the pores, the more plant material. If the pores are too small, some of the trichomes will not filter through.

3. COLLECT TRICHOMES

AFTER TRICHOMES ARE COLLECTED (HASH/KIEF)

DECARB/INFUSE

Cure over time or decarb following the same guidelines for flower. The least scent is curing over time. The quickest is in an oven.

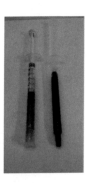

Infuse by heating and stirring into 20 ml carrier oil for an oral oil, or 1c/240ml for a topical oil.
(1oz/30g cannabis flower will make between .5 and 2 g hash or kief)

Strain with a coffee filter or super-fine mesh or cloth to filter the "skins" of the trichomes" if desired (not necessary).

This oil will be very light in color and taste mild in comparison to a FECO oil.

KIEF EXTRACT

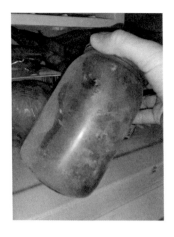

Freeze Plant Material

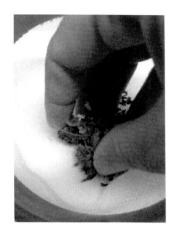

Rub Gently Over
Fine Mesh

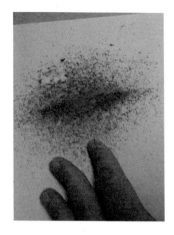

Collect Trichomes

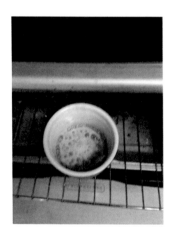

Decarb in Oven

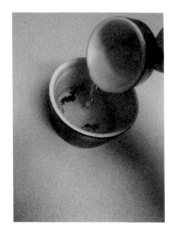

Add 20 ml Oil of Choice

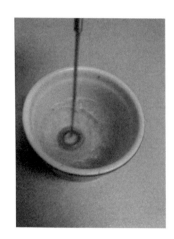

Stir/Whisk

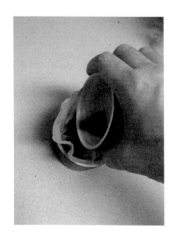

Filter

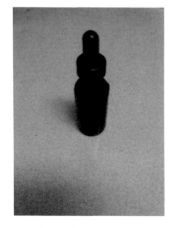

Pour into Bottle

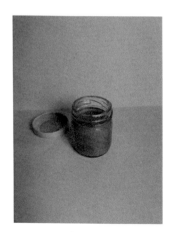

Or Jar

Tips and Tricks

Blending the flower before extraction is not necessary but recommended. It simply reduces the volume of cannabis in order to use less alcohol or oil.

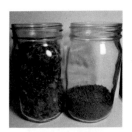

Heating either a solvent or an oil in a crockpot is easy and takes less attention than a stovetop. If the amount is too small to put in a larger crockpot, place ingredients in a glass jar and put the entire jar inside the crockpot with a lid on loosely (avoids alcohol from evaporating or water condensation from getting into an oil).

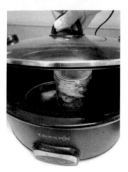

Food grade ingredients are always recommended

Add lecithin for slight thickening and to help the body use cannabinoids more efficiently.[5]

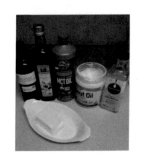

When straining, squeeze as much as possible for efficient use of the cannabis. Use 2 plates on a counter for more leverage. Other home tools may include a coffee press or a bench vice. Optional: Rinse strained material with alcohol and strain again.

The smaller the pores of the mesh strainer, the more plant material is removed. A coffee filter or fine microscreen you purchase online will filter the most and also take the longest to filter. Most of the time a cheesecloth or pillowcase is sufficient for at home use.

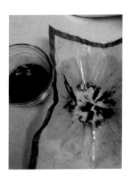

[5]Zgair, Atheer. "Dietary fats and pharmaceutical lipid excipients increase systemic exposure to orally administered cannabis" Am J Trans Res 2016 8(8) 3448-3459
https://www.ncbi.nlm.nih.gov/pmc/articles/PMC5009397

Larger Batches

If you plan to make larger (more than 30g/1oz) more frequent batches, it may be useful to invest in some specialized equipment.

The Magical Butter Machine has a built in blender, 4 heat settings including no heat, and 4 time settings. It can be plugged in and left safely. This machine can be used for both alcohol and oils. (If using heat and alcohol, it is best to monitor in person).

To save on the cost of alcohol for larger or more frequent batches, consider using a countertop distiller. It is generally sold as water distiller since making alcohol is illegal in many places. After straining the flower material, this machine will "reclaim" up to 70% of the alcohol by heating it into vapor and then re-condensing it into a container. It **should** have a fan built in so the alcohol fumes do not build up inside.

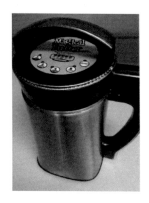 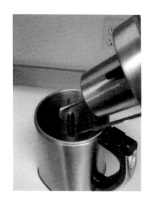 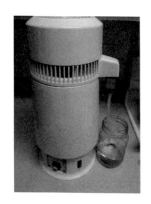

ADVANCED SOLVENT CONCEPT: Winterizing/Clarifying

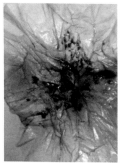

Alcohol also extracts the plant waxes. This adds to the taste, color, and volume of a Full Extract Cannabis Oil (FECO). There is no need to remove these waxes for oral, sublingual, and topical uses. However, retail producers (and those inhaling oil), remove these waxes. It clarifies the oil and, for some, tastes less bitter.

After straining the cannabis (Step 2 in **Solvent**), freeze the alcohol solution for at least a day. For each cup of solution, rubberband a coffee filter (or other fine filter) over a mason jar. Quickly remove the solution from the freezer and pour into the filters allowing solution to drip into jars. Remove the rubberband and squeeze the remaining alcohol through the filter to remove the frozen waxes. Continue to evaporate as described previously (p.18).

How to Use Cannabis (Methods of Delivery)

In addition to the strain, (chemotype/genotype), **how cannabis is used can alter its effect in the body.** There is no right (or wrong) way to use cannabis. All methods are useful. Often a combination of applications if most effective.

Topical: *Salve/balm/lotion*: External use on skin.

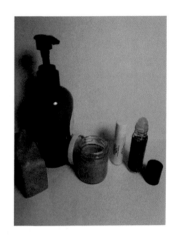

- Useful for beginners
- Apply directly to the area of discomfort
- May absorb through skin into the bloodstream[6]
- Common uses: tremors (rub on arms/legs), aches, sore muscles, nausea (rub directly on stomach), back pain, headaches, lung infections (rub directly on chest), psoriasis, eczema, acne, melanomas, skin cancer, cuts, scrapes, bruises, fibromyalgia, a general sense of calm

Oral: *Oil/edible:* Taken internally through mouth or G-tube

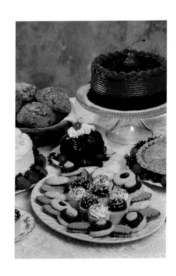

- Processed in stomach; enters bloodstream in 1-3 hours
- **First-pass metabolism** sends nutrients (cannabinoids) to be processed by the liver before entering the bloodstream. (Versus other methods of entering the bloodstream directly and bypassing the liver initially). The liver processes cannabinoids and produces different chemicals (11-hydroxy-THC) which create different effects. This explains why an edible THC makes a "body high" much stronger for many individuals than a similar sublingual dose.
- Common uses: any stomach or digestive issues, cancers, nausea, pain, Crohn's, full body condition

---

[6] Huestis, Marilyn. "Human Cannabinoid Pharmacokinetics." Chem Biodivers 2007 Aug 4(8) 1770-1804. https://www.ncbi.nlm.nih.gov/pmc/articles/PMC2689518/

Sublingual: *Oil/tincture:* Taken under tongue by spray or drops

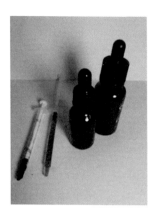

- Enters bloodstream in 1-15 minutes
- Avoids liver first-pass processing, which is useful if
    - taking other medications
    - genetic mutations or dysfunction in liver
    - do not like effects of oral THC
- quick delivery in emergency (ex: seizure)
- Common uses: Seizures, nerve pain, neurological diagnosis, fibromyalgia, autism, ADHD.

Suppository: *Capsule:* Inserted into vagina or rectum.

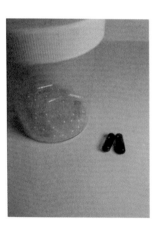

- Enters bloodstream 1-15 minutes
- Use higher dose of THC with less psychoactive effect
- Anyone unable to dose using other methods
- Common uses: cervical or ovarian cancers, vaginitis, rectal, colon, or prostate cancers, any illness related to/or in the area of the uterus, rectum, colon, intestines.

Transdermal Patch: *Bandage on skin*

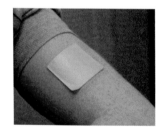

- Considered "medical device"
- Delivers medicine over time
- Not common
- A homemade patch can be used with a topical solution, but it would not be defined "transdermal" unless it was able to deliver a set dose over time.
- Usually produced in a lab.

Making products to Inhale is not covered in this manual. For reference here are the methods of inhaling available in legal areas.

Inhaler or Nebulizer: *Direct to lungs*

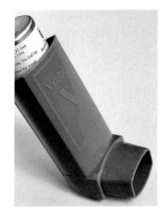

- Enters bloodstream in 1-15 minutes
- Bypasses liver initially
- Typically available in a dispensary setting
- Increasingly popular for older children and teens with ADD, Autism, and other diagnosis with difficult emotions and behaviors

Vaporizer/Vape Pen: *Direct to lungs*

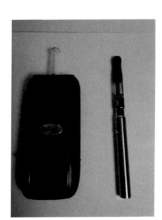

- Enters bloodstream in 1-15 minutes
- Vaporizer raises the temperature of cannabis flower or oil to turn cannabinoids into vapor.
- Avoids inhaling smoke from the plant material
- Can be an expectorant
- Common uses: pain, anxiety, depression, COPD, emphysema and *same as above.*

Pipe/Joint: *Direct to lungs.*

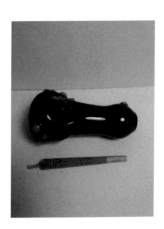

- Smoked as flower
- Not highly recommended for medically frail patients
- Can be an expectorant
- Common uses: recreational, anxiety, depression, pain

Dosing

Pharmaceutical Dosing

Pharmaceutical versions of cannabis usually add or subtract
cannabinoids (and terpenes). The solution (carrier) is another
lab chemical. These changes may affect the success of
cannabis in the body.

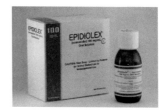

Cannabis medications are prescribed like similar pharmaceuticals. Often based on body
weight and increased over a few weeks (titrated) until a "working" dose is reached. For
example: Epidiolex begins at 5mg CBD/kg/day increasing to 10mg CBD/kg/day. For a
55 lb child this is **125mg per day** to start and 250mg to maintain.

Herbal Dosing

Herbal dosing is based on the amount of the plant material, or oil.
Each component of the whole plant works together in symbiosis
with the body. The carrier oil helps the body absorb the nutrients.

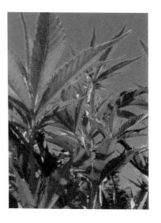

A personal recommended dilution (as outlined in Methods of
Extraction) is 1ml FECO to 20 ml carrier oil. A beginning dose is
one drop (1/20th of a ml). Rarely exceeding 4 drops. **A daily
dose averages 2-12-mg** depending on the strain. A significant
difference from a pharmaceutical dose.

Microdosing is the concept of using a small amount of cannabis all of the time in order
to avoid building tolerance. I think of this like a vitamin that stimulates the body to do
what it needs instead of overpowering it. (However, an extremely diluted preparation
may not even have 1mg of CBD per ml. See Calculating A Dose p.37.) The dose is
small regardless of body weight (adults and children use same dose).

 Changing a strain may be useful if a preparation does not help anymore.

Dispensary Dosing   In dispensaries, a "dose" is often 5-10mg of THC or CBD.

Epilepsy Considerations

The cannabis legalization movement gained momentum when parents began using high CBD oil for children with intractable epilepsy.

CBD is the most studied and used cannabinoid in epilepsy. However, for many patients CBD or "Hemp" oil is not enough. Strains with 1% - >20% THC can be more effective depending on the seizure type and individual.

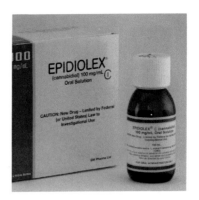

High THC strains can work as a rescue medication and are useful while weaning medications when withdrawal seizures and other symptoms are at a peak.

Microdosing using an herbal philosophy makes the most sense to me at this time. Specifics listed on previous page. I give our child 2 drops of a solution made with 1 ml FECO and 20 ml carrier oil. This is approximately 3-6 mg CBD per day. I use the same dilution ratio for each batch so it is easier to switch strains.

Because Anti-Epileptic Drugs (AED) and cannabis are usually **all metabolized in the p450 cytochrome system**, it is necessary to take them at different times so they enter the bloodstream separately.

Taking cannabis sublingual avoids first pass metabolism in the liver.

A patient taking <u>only cannabis</u> does not need to worry about interactions or as many potential adverse effects. Missing a dose <u>does not</u> increase the likelihood of a seizure, whereas skipping an AED will most likely cause a seizure (possibly status).

I highly recommend getting a p450 genetics test before ANY pharmaceutical is used . This test will identify an individual's genetic predisposition to metabolizing medications. Although the results do not currently include cannabis, the genes listed can easily be researched to determine whether CBD, THC or other cannabinoids will be effective in an individual's body and how they will react with other medications. See Resources (p.42) for additional information.

All are opinions based on personal experience

Cancer Considerations

Cannabis can be used in a variety of ways to help with cancer treatment.

Many people use **cannabis In conjunction** with typical treatments of radiation or chemo to alleviate nausea, pain, and depression.

Others choose cannabis as the cancer treatment. A protocol was developed by cancer survivor and cannabis advocate Rick Simpson. FECO is ingested starting with a very small dose and increasing to a dose of 1mg per day for 60 days. More info is available on his website www.phoenixtears.ca.

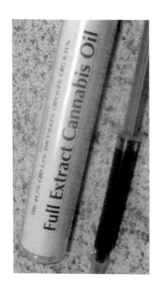

Many educators take this basic formula and adapt it to their beliefs and needs. Some people may respond successfully with only half of the recommended dose. Some may need more. A "dose" can be measured by tolerance. When increasing tolerance, stop when the patient begins to feel "high" regularly without adapting to the increased dose. This maximum dose can be considered the "working dose" for the 60 day time frame. Some prefer to continue the dose for 90 days.

In the past, patients used high THC strains. However, with the availability of high CBD strains, more patients are experimenting with different chemotypes. Studies are popping up daily in an effort to study these strains in cancer treatments.

Cancers fed by estrogen seem to also be fed by THC. CBD counters this effect and stops the cancer from metastasizing.[7] It is suggested by cannabis educators to use equal parts THC and CBD (1:1), **or** high CBD strains in estrogen-fed cancers or other cancers as preferred. Currently, a few patients are also experimenting with CBDA to stop and eliminate cancer.

Each individual responds in a unique way.

---

[7] McAllister, MD. "Pathways mediating the effects of cannabidiol on the effects of breast cancer cell proliferation, invasion, and metastasis." Breast Cancer Res Treat 2011 Aug 129 (1) 37-47 https://www.ncbi.nlm.nih.gov/pubmed/20859676

Testing

It is certainly not necessary to test. People have been successfully using cannabis medicinally for centuries with no testing available. But in certain circumstances, it may be useful. Growers may want to confirm a strain, a consumer may want to verify a purchase, an oil maker may want to have a better idea of the concentration, etc.

In legal areas, testing may be easily accessed and affordable. A lab can test for pesticides, cannabinoids, terpenes, mold, and even genetics. There are also expensive pieces of equipment that scan and validate through an app on your phone. I am not familiar with the outcomes of these products.

Thin Layer Chromatography is a relatively inexpensive testing method that can be used at home. It visualizes the cannabinoids in a flower, oil, or other sample. I use this personally to confirm the potency of flower and oils I make.

Identified cannabinoids include:

CBD
THC
THCV
CBG
CBC

ACIDS
CBDA
THCA
CBGA
CBCA

These tests are useful to see how many cannabinoids have been decarbed.

In this photo, the 3rd and 4th samples have a large amount of cannabinoids that are still in the acid form. These flowers or oils can be decarbed (heated) longer if the intention is to get more THC or CBD.

If the intention is to have a full range of all cannabinoids including acids, then these are perfect.

Different decarb methods may show slightly different fingerprints.

Plants can be tested in any stage of growth using fan leaves for growers wanting to verify the basic cannabinoids present.

Comparing Different Products

It may be useful (though not necessary) to know an **approximate** amount of cannabinoids in a product. Knowing how to read a label or test result is useful for dosing, switching products or simply comparing value. **One milliliter of oil A might have the same amount of cannabinoids as an entire bottle of oil B. One drop of oil A may be the same dose as 2ml of oil B.** Calculating an exact amount does not mean the body is using that exact amount. Estimating whether a product contains a high, medium, or low amount of cannabinoids is sufficient.

CANNABINOID GUIDELINES (THC OR CBD OR COMBO):

FLOWER:	High: 20-29%	Medium: 15-20%	Low:10-15%	
FECO:	High: >75%	Medium: 50-70%	Low: 30-50%	
DILUTED:	High:6-10%	Medium: 3-5%	Low: 1-3%	SuperLow: >1%

**(Add a "0" to get mg/ml as described on the next page)

Most store-bought products have a label indicating the amount of cannabinoids. Sometimes acids and their counterparts are listed separately. Sometimes a product that has clearly not been decarbed only lists THC. This is not possible since there will be acids in a flower. Many labs use an equation (THCA x .877= THC) in order to estimate the THC that will be available after decarb. Ask questions to make sure what the label says is understood.

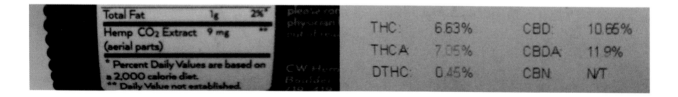

Common ways to express cannabinoid content on a label include percentage, ratio, milligram per bottle, milligram per milliliter.

In order to **effectively compare** products, cannabinoids need to be in the same unit of measurement. I prefer **milligram of the cannabinoid per milliliter (mg/ml).**

FOR ALL LIQUID AND OIL CALCULATIONS: 1 gram = 1 milliliter

If the product is expressed in percent:

Convert percent to mg.

Example: 17% THC in 1g Flower

$17/100 = X/1000$
$.17 \times 1000 = X$
$170 = X$ There is 170 mg of THC in 1 g flower

Shortcut: Remove the percent sign and add a 0

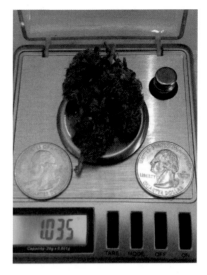

Flower potency is always expressed in percent. Other products may use percent. A percent is the amount of the cannabinoid per **GRAM**. A gram of flower looks like this

If the product is expressed in mg per bottle:

Divide the mg of THC by the number of ml in the bottle (1 oz = 30 ml)

Example: There are 54 mg of THC in this 2 oz (60ml) jar. How many mg of THC per ml?

$54 / 60 = .9$

Approximately 1 mg of THC per mL

If a product is expressed in ratio :

A ratio simply shows how much an oil has compared to another oil. It DOES NOT indicate the amount of cannabinoids in a product. These bottles should also include at least one testing number.
(Exception: see resources)

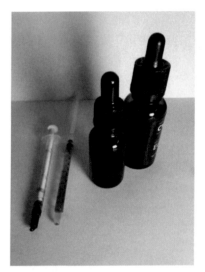

One gram of FECO is the same as 1 ml. Adding oil dilutes the potency for dosing. See dilution equation.

Examples: 1:1 THC: CBD   1:2 CBD: THC   3:2 CBD:THC

Calculate one cannabinoid using other methods and then multiply or divide to determine the other cannabinoid.

If the product is being diluted or extracted into another form:

Sometimes a consumer will buy flower or FECO from a dispensary and make a different product. In order to estimate how many cannabinoids are in the new product, a dilution equation can be used even if it is being concentrated! (ex: making FECO with flower).

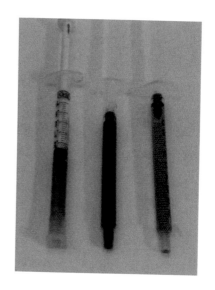

Dilution equation

- **C1**=concentration of **original** solution in mg/g (convert from percent)
- **V1**=volume of original solution
- **C2**=concentration of new solution
- **V2**=volume of new solution

C1 x V1 = C2 x V2

Plug in what is known to estimate the new solution.

Example:

Consumer buys 1 gram (1 mL) of 75% FECO and wants to add a carrier oil to make it easier to use. Consumer mixes the FECO with one ounce (30mL) of coconut oil.

C1= 750
C2= X
V1= 1g
V2=30mL

$$750 \, x \, 1 = X \, x \, 30$$
$$750 \, / \, 30 = X$$
$$25 = X$$

New solution has 25 mg THC per mL
(To calculate average per drop divide by 20. A 1ml syringe has approximately 20 drops).

Purchasing Cannabis

If you do not grow your own, you will be purchasing a premade product, flower, FECO, or hash to make oil. Due to local laws, it is common in many dispensaries to distinguish *"medical"* cannabis from *"recreational"* cannabis

In order to understand the terminology and certain preferences, it is easier to distinguish "smoking" users from "non-smoking" users. Or **Inhale vs Ingest.**

Those inhaling cannabis (ex: smoking or vaping), have different standards of appearance and presentation. Retail products have certain standards to meet. Keep this in mind when determining why one product may be "superior" to another.

Inhale

Qualities that may be important to someone inhaling include visual appearance, smell, amount of trichomes on a flower, color of the extract, percent of THC.

It is often important that "impurities" are removed for a product that is inhaled. These are typically plant waxes and/or chlorophyll. These "impurities" are not harmful in a product that is ingested.

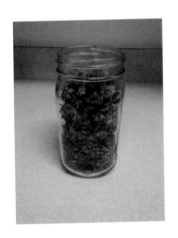

Ingest

Qualities important to ingesting may be high quality food grade or organic ingredients, taste, flavorings, percent of THC or CBD, method of extraction.

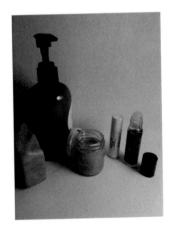

Ordering CBD or Hemp Oil Online

Hemp and CBD products have quickly become a worldwide industry. Currently, there are no clear labeling requirements. Sometimes a company is uneducated about cannabis concepts presented in this guide. The public only knows what is advertised. The previous discussion on Hemp Confusion (p.9) may help clarify these misunderstandings. Products can be mistakenly labeled and marketed as CBD or Hemp oil when in fact it may be Hemp Seed Oil. Other products may combine CBDA and CBD into one reported number (CBD).

Helpful hints:

Look for cannabinoid content or mg of CBD on the label

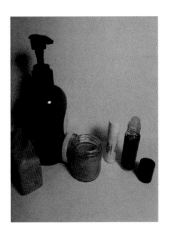

Calculate amount of milligrams of CBD per milliliter to compare value.

Choose a local company with reputable owners. There are several companies in the USA founded by parents and caregivers of children with epilepsy. These owners are well educated and use top quality ingredients and extraction methods.

If possible, call and speak with someone.

Many high CBD products are "isolates" or have THC and other cannabinoids removed. If searching for a "full extract" or "whole plant extract", it is best to find out how the product is processed before purchasing.

If a "hemp" CBD or "isolate" preparation is not effective, consider using a strain that has slightly more THC. Even 1% THC to 20% CBD may be more effective than "hemp" (.3%THC to 10-20%CBD). These strengths are currently only found in legal locations around the world.

Resources

The Wild Weed www.thewildweed.com for videos to these processes

Cannabinoid test kit www.theweedtest.com

Pesticide test kit www.anphealth.com

Magical Butter Machine www.magicalbutter.com Use code **thewildweed** for $25 off

Reclaim unit www.amazon.com or www.ebay.com any water distiller with a fan

Decarboxylating chamber www.ardent.com

Organic Alcohol www.organicalcohol.com

P450 testing https://genesight.com/ or as recommended by healthcare professional

High CBD/Hemp Oil Available in the USA founded for children with epilepsy. All have similar amounts of cannabinoids per ml for legal reasons, yet have more than the majority of Super-Low products sold online. All use the whole plant.

Charlotte's Web https://www.charlottesweb.com/ (solvent method alcohol and CO2)
Hailey's Hope https://haleighshope.com/products/ (solvent method CO2)
Palmetto Harmony https://palmettoharmony.com/ (infusion method)

Made in the USA
Middletown, DE
06 July 2019